Diabetes Wellness:

Nourish and Thrive

Dr. Adam West

©2022 All Rights Reserved.

No part of this book may be reproduced, distributed or transmitted in any form or by any means including electronic, mechanical, photocopying, recording or by any information storehouse and reclamation system, without written permission from the author, except for the additional brief citations in a review

This book is dedicated to my Late Sister, Olivia. You have been my source of strength in this journey till date.

Catalog

Chapter 1: Understanding Diabetes

Introduction to Diabetes and its Impact on Health:

Diabetes, a chronic metabolic disorder, has emerged as a significant health concern worldwide, affecting millions of lives and necessitating a deeper understanding of its intricacies. At its core, diabetes is characterized by the body's inability to effectively regulate blood sugar levels, leading to elevated glucose concentrations in the bloodstream. This condition arises due to insufficient insulin production, impaired insulin utilization, or a combination of both.

Insulin, a hormone produced by the pancreas, plays a pivotal role in glucose metabolism. It acts as a key that unlocks cells, allowing them to absorb glucose from the blood for energy. In individuals with diabetes, this finely tuned system falters. Type 1 diabetes results from the immune system attacking and destroying insulin-producing beta cells, leaving the body reliant on external insulin. On the other hand, Type 2 diabetes often stems from insulin resistance, where cells fail to respond adequately to insulin, and the pancreas struggles to produce enough to compensate.

The impact of diabetes on health extends beyond fluctuations in blood sugar levels. Uncontrolled diabetes can give rise to a cascade of complications, affecting various organs and systems in the body. High blood sugar levels can damage blood vessels, leading to cardiovascular complications such as heart disease and stroke. Additionally, the kidneys may face strain, potentially resulting in chronic kidney disease. Nerve damage, known as neuropathy, can manifest, causing pain, tingling, and numbness in extremities.

The eyes are not immune to the effects of diabetes, with diabetic retinopathy posing a risk to vision. Poorly managed diabetes can also compromise the immune system, making individuals more susceptible to infections. Foot problems, including ulcers and infections, can arise due to impaired circulation and nerve damage.

Furthermore, diabetes intersects with other health conditions, creating a complex web of challenges. For instance, the relationship between diabetes and obesity is well-established, as excess body weight contributes to insulin resistance. Diabetes management becomes a critical aspect of overall health, emphasizing the need for a comprehensive and proactive approach.

Understanding the impact of diabetes on health underscores the importance of effective management strategies. Beyond the immediate concern of blood sugar control, individuals must embrace lifestyle changes, nutrition choices, and regular monitoring to mitigate the risk of complications. A holistic approach to diabetes care not only enhances physical well-being but also fosters a higher quality of life, empowering individuals to navigate the complexities of this condition with resilience and knowledge.

Types of diabetes and their distinctions

Understanding the different types of diabetes is crucial for effective management and tailored treatment plans. Broadly, diabetes can be categorized into three main types: Type 1 diabetes, Type 2 diabetes, and gestational diabetes.

1. Type 1 Diabetes:
Type 1 diabetes is an autoimmune condition where the immune system mistakenly attacks and destroys the insulin-producing beta cells in the pancreas. This results in a lack of insulin, the hormone responsible for regulating blood sugar levels. Typically diagnosed in childhood or adolescence, individuals with Type 1 diabetes require lifelong insulin therapy for survival. The exact cause of this autoimmune response is not fully understood, but both genetic and environmental factors are believed to play a role. Managing Type 1 diabetes involves regular insulin injections or the use of an insulin pump, coupled with close monitoring of blood sugar levels.

2. Type 2 Diabetes:
Type 2 diabetes is the most common form of diabetes, accounting for the majority of cases worldwide. Unlike Type 1 diabetes, individuals with Type 2 diabetes produce insulin, but their bodies either do not use it effectively (insulin resistance) or do not produce enough insulin to meet the body's needs. This form of diabetes is

often associated with lifestyle factors, including poor dietary habits, sedentary behavior, and obesity. While it can develop at any age, Type 2 diabetes is more commonly diagnosed in adulthood. Initially, lifestyle modifications such as diet and exercise may be sufficient to manage Type 2 diabetes, but medication or insulin therapy may be necessary as the condition progresses.

3. Gestational Diabetes:
Gestational diabetes occurs during pregnancy when the body is unable to produce enough insulin to meet the increased demands. This condition can lead to complications for both the mother and the baby. While gestational diabetes typically resolves after childbirth, women who have experienced it are at an increased risk of developing Type 2 diabetes later in life. Managing gestational diabetes involves close monitoring of blood sugar levels, dietary adjustments, and, in some cases, insulin therapy to ensure the health of both mother and baby.

In addition to these main types, there are also less common forms of diabetes, such as monogenic diabetes and secondary diabetes, which result from specific genetic conditions or other medical conditions, respectively. Understanding the distinctions between these types of diabetes is crucial for healthcare professionals to provide personalized care and empower individuals to manage their condition effectively.

Importance of blood sugar control for overall well-being

Maintaining optimal blood sugar levels is paramount for overall well-being, and it plays a crucial role in supporting various bodily functions. The importance of blood sugar control extends far beyond managing diabetes; it is a fundamental aspect of general health and vitality.

1. Energy Regulation:
   Balanced blood sugar levels are essential for regulating energy production in the body. Glucose, derived from the breakdown of carbohydrates, serves as the primary source of energy for cells. Consistent blood sugar control ensures a steady supply of glucose to cells, promoting sustained energy levels throughout the day.

2. Brain Function:

The brain is highly sensitive to fluctuations in blood sugar levels. Maintaining stable glucose concentrations is vital for cognitive functions such as concentration, memory, and decision-making. Unstable blood sugar levels can contribute to mood swings, difficulty focusing, and mental fatigue.

3. Mood Stability:
   Blood sugar imbalances can influence mood and emotional well-being. Rapid spikes and crashes in blood sugar levels may contribute to irritability, anxiety, and feelings of lethargy. Stable blood sugar levels, on the other hand, support a more consistent and positive mood.

4. Weight Management:
   Effective blood sugar control is closely linked to weight management. Elevated blood sugar levels can lead to increased fat storage, especially around the abdomen. By regulating blood sugar, the body is better equipped to manage weight, reducing the risk of obesity and related health issues.

5. Cardiovascular Health:
   Prolonged high blood sugar levels can contribute to cardiovascular complications. It may lead to damage to blood vessels, increasing the risk of

heart disease, stroke, and other circulatory issues. Maintaining blood sugar within a healthy range supports overall cardiovascular well-being.

6. Prevention of Diabetes Complications:
   For individuals with diabetes, consistent blood sugar control is crucial for preventing long-term complications. These complications include kidney disease, vision problems, nerve damage, and cardiovascular issues. Proper management helps minimize the risk of these complications and enhances overall quality of life.

7. Enhanced Immune Function:
   Stable blood sugar levels contribute to a robust immune system. Fluctuations in glucose can compromise immune function, making the body more susceptible to infections and illnesses. By keeping blood sugar in check, the immune system is better equipped to defend against pathogens.

8. Reduced Risk of Hypoglycemia:
   Maintaining blood sugar control helps prevent episodes of hypoglycemia (low blood sugar), which can lead to dizziness, confusion, and, in severe cases, unconsciousness. Consistent blood sugar levels contribute to a more stable and safe physiological state.

In conclusion, the importance of blood sugar control extends across various facets of health, influencing energy levels, cognitive function, emotional well-being, weight management, cardiovascular health, and immune function. Whether managing diabetes or aiming for general health optimization, maintaining stable blood sugar levels is a foundational element of overall well-being.

Chapter 2: Nutrition Essentials

Fundamentals of a balanced diabetic-friendly diet

A balanced diabetic-friendly diet is a cornerstone of effective diabetes management, designed to regulate blood sugar levels and promote overall health. At its core, this dietary approach emphasizes the consumption of nutrient-dense foods while carefully managing the intake of carbohydrates, particularly those with a high glycemic index. Here, we delve into the fundamental principles of crafting a diet that aligns with the needs of individuals living with diabetes.

Central to a diabetic-friendly diet is the concept of carbohydrate control. Carbohydrates have a direct impact on blood sugar levels, and managing their intake is crucial for stabilizing glucose levels. Rather than focusing solely on avoiding carbohydrates, the emphasis is placed on choosing complex carbohydrates with a lower glycemic index. These include whole grains, legumes, and vegetables, which release glucose more gradually, preventing rapid spikes in blood sugar.

In addition to carbohydrates, the diet should incorporate lean proteins, which play a vital role in satiety, muscle maintenance, and blood sugar regulation. Sources of lean protein include poultry, fish, tofu, legumes, and low-fat dairy products. Protein-rich foods contribute to a balanced and satisfying diet, helping individuals manage their weight effectively.

Healthy fats also feature prominently in a diabetic-friendly diet. While moderation is key, including sources of monounsaturated and polyunsaturated fats, such as avocados, nuts, seeds, and olive oil, can provide essential nutrients without adversely affecting blood sugar levels. These fats contribute to heart health and help individuals feel satisfied after meals.

Vegetables, particularly non-starchy varieties, are essential components of a balanced diabetic-friendly diet. Rich in fiber, vitamins, and minerals, vegetables contribute to overall well-being and assist in maintaining steady blood sugar levels.

Dark leafy greens, colorful peppers, and cruciferous vegetables are valuable additions that enhance the nutritional profile of meals.

Portion control is another fundamental aspect of a diabetic-friendly diet. Monitoring portion sizes helps regulate calorie intake, preventing overconsumption and promoting weight management. This approach allows individuals to enjoy a variety of foods while maintaining control over their overall energy balance.

Regular monitoring of blood sugar levels is essential for individuals with diabetes, and the dietary plan should be flexible to accommodate these fluctuations. Being mindful of how different foods affect blood sugar empowers individuals to make informed choices and adapt their diet to their unique needs.

Ultimately, a balanced diabetic-friendly diet is not about restriction but rather about making thoughtful and informed choices. It empowers individuals to enjoy a diverse range of nutrient-dense foods, supporting their overall health while effectively managing blood sugar levels. By embracing these fundamentals, individuals with diabetes can cultivate a sustainable and nourishing approach to eating that enhances their well-being and quality of life.

Exploring macronutrients and their role in diabetes management

In the intricate landscape of diabetes management, understanding macronutrients and their nuanced roles is pivotal for individuals striving to maintain optimal blood sugar levels. Macronutrients, comprising carbohydrates, proteins, and fats, form the foundation of our dietary intake and exert profound effects on the body's metabolism. Delving into the intricate interplay of these macronutrients is essential for crafting a tailored dietary strategy in the context of diabetes.

Carbohydrates, often regarded as the primary player in diabetes nutrition, have a direct impact on blood sugar levels. The body breaks down carbohydrates into glucose, influencing blood glucose levels. For individuals with diabetes, the focus is on managing the type and quantity of carbohydrates consumed. Embracing complex carbohydrates, found in whole grains, legumes, and vegetables, provides a gradual release of glucose, preventing abrupt spikes. Portion control becomes paramount, allowing for a balanced intake that aligns with individual glycemic responses.

Proteins assume a multifaceted role in diabetes management. Apart from their crucial contribution to muscle maintenance and repair, proteins also influence satiety and blood sugar regulation. Including lean protein sources, such as poultry, fish, tofu, and legumes, helps stabilize blood sugar levels while promoting a sense of fullness. Striking a balance between protein intake and other macronutrients is pivotal, fostering a well-rounded and satisfying dietary profile.

Fats, often misconceived in the context of diabetes, play a vital role in metabolic health. Opting for healthy fats, such as monounsaturated and polyunsaturated fats found in avocados, nuts, seeds, and olive oil, contributes to cardiovascular well-being without negatively impacting blood sugar levels. The emphasis lies in moderation and choosing sources that align with heart health goals, establishing a harmonious relationship between dietary fats and diabetes management.

Understanding the synergy between these macronutrients becomes especially crucial during meal planning. Striking a delicate balance ensures sustained energy release, mitigates blood sugar fluctuations, and supports overall metabolic health. This holistic approach involves not only selecting nutrient-dense foods but also considering the timing and combination of macronutrients in meals.

Moreover, the glycemic index (GI) serves as a valuable tool in navigating carbohydrate choices. Integrating low-GI foods into the diet helps individuals manage blood sugar more effectively. This nuanced understanding of macronutrients empowers individuals with diabetes to make informed decisions, promoting dietary flexibility without compromising metabolic control.

In essence, exploring macronutrients in the context of diabetes management transcends mere nutritional awareness; it encapsulates a comprehensive understanding of how each component contributes to the intricate dance of metabolic regulation. Armed with this knowledge, individuals can embark on a dietary journey that not only aligns with their health goals but also cultivates a sustainable and nourishing approach to living with diabetes.

Portion control and mindful eating practices

Portion control and mindful eating practices constitute a profound and transformative approach to nutrition, offering individuals, particularly those managing diabetes, a gateway to fostering a harmonious relationship with food. Far beyond mere measurements on a plate, these practices encompass a holistic understanding of hunger cues, satiety signals, and the sensory experience of eating, creating a mindful awareness that extends beyond the act of consumption.

Portion control emerges as a pivotal aspect of diabetes management, serving as a linchpin for regulating caloric intake and, subsequently, blood sugar levels. It involves the conscious moderation of portion sizes to align with individual energy needs. By adhering to recommended serving sizes, individuals can avoid overconsumption, a crucial consideration in maintaining a healthy weight, which is intimately linked to diabetes management.

However, portion control is not about deprivation or rigid constraints; rather, it encourages a nuanced approach to enjoying a diverse array of foods in appropriate amounts. This practice allows individuals to savor the flavors and textures of meals while cultivating a keen awareness of their body's nutritional requirements.

Mindful eating, on the other hand, transcends the quantitative aspect of portion control and delves into the qualitative experience of eating. It involves being present and fully engaged during meals, savoring each bite, and appreciating the sensory aspects of the dining experience. For individuals with diabetes, mindful eating introduces a heightened awareness of how different foods impact blood sugar levels and satiety.

Mindful eating encourages individuals to listen to their bodies, recognizing hunger and fullness cues. By paying attention to internal signals rather than external influences, such as societal expectations or emotional triggers, individuals can develop a more intuitive and responsive relationship with food. This attunement to the body's cues supports better blood sugar control, as meals are consumed in a manner that aligns with the body's metabolic needs.

Moreover, mindful eating promotes a sense of enjoyment and satisfaction from meals, fostering a positive relationship with food. By engaging all senses in the act of eating, individuals can derive more pleasure from their meals, potentially reducing the likelihood of overindulgence driven by emotional or external factors.

In the context of diabetes, these practices synergize to create a holistic approach to nutrition that goes beyond mere dietary restrictions. Portion control and mindful eating, when integrated into daily life, empower individuals to make conscious and informed choices, establishing a sustainable and enjoyable foundation for diabetes management. Through these practices, individuals can navigate the intricate landscape of nutrition with a sense of balance, mindfulness, and a deeper connection to the nourishing qualities of the food they consume.

Chapter 3: Mastering the Glycemic Index

Demystifying the glycemic index and its significance

Demystifying the glycemic index (GI) unravels a fundamental aspect of nutrition, particularly pertinent for individuals managing diabetes. The glycemic index is a tool that classifies carbohydrates based on their potential to raise blood sugar levels. By understanding the significance of this index, individuals can make informed choices about the types of carbohydrates they include in their diet, ultimately contributing to better blood sugar control and overall health.

At its essence, the glycemic index is a numerical scale that ranks carbohydrates on a scale from 0 to 100, with each value representing how quickly a specific food increases blood sugar levels when compared to a reference food, usually pure glucose. Foods with a high glycemic index are rapidly digested and cause a quick spike in blood sugar, while those with a low glycemic index are absorbed more slowly, resulting in a gradual and more controlled rise in blood sugar.

The significance of the glycemic index lies in its ability to guide individuals toward choosing carbohydrates that have a gentler impact on blood sugar levels. For people with diabetes, this knowledge is paramount as it helps in managing their condition by preventing sharp fluctuations in blood glucose, which can be detrimental to their health.

High-GI foods, such as white bread, sugary cereals, and certain processed snacks, are swiftly broken down into glucose, leading to rapid spikes in blood sugar. In contrast, low-GI foods, like whole grains, legumes, and most vegetables, release glucose more gradually, providing a sustained and stable source of energy.

Moreover, understanding the glycemic index is not solely about categorizing foods but also about grasping the concept of glycemic load. The glycemic load takes into account both the quality and quantity of carbohydrates in a serving, offering a more comprehensive view of a food's impact on blood sugar. This nuanced approach allows individuals to consider not only the type of carbohydrate but also the portion size when making dietary choices.

Incorporating low-GI and moderate-GI foods into the diet can be particularly beneficial for individuals with diabetes. It enables them to enjoy a diverse range of nutrient-dense foods while promoting steady blood sugar levels. This knowledge empowers individuals to make choices that align with their specific dietary needs and preferences, providing a practical tool for navigating the complex landscape of diabetes management.

In essence, demystifying the glycemic index is about empowering individuals to make conscious and informed decisions about the carbohydrates they consume. By incorporating this understanding into their dietary habits, individuals can wield the glycemic index as a valuable ally in their quest for stable blood sugar levels, enhanced well-being, and a more nuanced approach to nutrition.

Using the glycemic load to make smarter food choices

Harnessing the glycemic load (GL) as a guiding principle in food choices represents a sophisticated approach to nutrition, particularly relevant for individuals, including those managing diabetes, seeking to navigate the intricate interplay between diet and blood sugar control. The glycemic load builds upon the foundation laid by the glycemic index, offering a more comprehensive perspective that considers both the quality and quantity of carbohydrates in a given serving.

Understanding the glycemic load involves recognizing that not all carbohydrates are created equal. While the glycemic index classifies foods based on their immediate impact on blood sugar, the glycemic load refines this concept by factoring in the amount of carbohydrates consumed. It is, in essence, a more nuanced metric that paints a fuller picture of a food's glycemic impact.

By incorporating the glycemic load into food choices, individuals can make smarter decisions about what to include in their diets. This approach is particularly valuable for those managing diabetes, as it empowers them to consider not only the type of carbohydrates but also the portion sizes, offering a more tailored and personalized strategy for blood sugar control.

High-glycemic-load foods, even if they have a moderate or low glycemic index, can contribute to significant spikes in blood sugar if consumed in large quantities. On the other hand, low-glycemic-load foods, even with a higher glycemic index, may have a gentler impact on blood sugar if consumed in appropriate portions. This nuanced understanding allows individuals to optimize their food choices based on both the quality and quantity of carbohydrates, creating a more flexible and sustainable approach to nutrition.

For instance, a small serving of watermelon, despite having a high glycemic index, may have a relatively low glycemic load due to its lower carbohydrate content per serving. This insight allows individuals to enjoy a variety of foods without being overly restricted, as long as they are mindful of portion sizes and the overall impact on blood sugar levels.

Furthermore, the glycemic load emphasizes the importance of balance in meal planning. Combining high-glycemic-load foods with those that have a lower glycemic load can help mitigate the overall impact on blood sugar. This strategic pairing fosters a more diverse and enjoyable diet, promoting not only blood sugar control but also overall well-being.

In essence, using the glycemic load to make smarter food choices transcends the simplistic categorization of foods. It invites individuals to engage with a deeper understanding of the nutritional composition of their meals, encouraging a mindful consideration of both the quality and quantity of carbohydrates. This approach empowers individuals, especially those managing diabetes, to craft a sustainable, individualized, and well-rounded dietary strategy that aligns with their health goals and fosters a positive relationship with food.

Incorporating low-GI foods into daily meals

Incorporating low glycemic index (GI) foods into daily meals emerges as a strategic and health-conscious approach to nutrition, offering a spectrum of benefits for individuals seeking to manage blood sugar levels, enhance satiety, and foster overall well-being. This dietary strategy involves selecting foods that have a lower impact on blood sugar, contributing to more stable glucose levels throughout the day.

At its core, the concept of the glycemic index classifies foods based on how quickly they cause a rise in blood sugar after consumption. Low-GI foods, characterized by a slower and more gradual release of glucose, play a pivotal role in creating a balanced and sustainable diet. By incorporating these foods into daily meals, individuals can harness their unique properties to optimize metabolic health.

The selection of low-GI foods encompasses a diverse range of options, including whole grains like quinoa and barley, legumes such as lentils and chickpeas, non-starchy vegetables like leafy greens and broccoli, and certain fruits like berries and apples. These choices not only provide essential nutrients but also contribute to a feeling of fullness and satisfaction, making them valuable components of a well-rounded meal.

In practical terms, integrating low-GI foods into daily meals involves thoughtful meal planning and a conscientious approach to food selection. For example, opting for whole grain alternatives instead of refined grains, choosing sweet potatoes over white potatoes, and incorporating a variety of colorful vegetables can significantly impact the overall glycemic profile of a meal.

This dietary strategy is particularly advantageous for individuals managing conditions like diabetes. By favoring low-GI foods, they can help regulate blood sugar levels, reducing the risk of sudden spikes and crashes that may accompany higher-GI choices. This becomes especially relevant during mealtime, where the careful selection of carbohydrates can influence post-meal glucose responses.

Beyond its impact on blood sugar, incorporating low-GI foods into daily meals contributes to sustained energy levels. The gradual release of glucose from these foods provides a stable source of fuel for the body, supporting physical activity, mental focus, and overall vitality throughout the day.

Furthermore, this approach aligns with broader health goals, promoting weight management and reducing the risk of chronic conditions associated with erratic blood sugar levels. The fiber content in many low-GI foods not only aids in digestion but also helps control appetite, contributing to a more mindful and balanced approach to eating.

In essence, incorporating low-GI foods into daily meals transcends a mere dietary choice; it represents a strategic and holistic approach to nutrition. By understanding the glycemic impact of different foods and intentionally selecting those with a lower GI, individuals can actively shape their diets to support metabolic health, enhance overall well-being, and cultivate a sustainable and enjoyable relationship with food.

Chapter 4: Building Diabetic-Friendly Meals

Recipe ideas and meal planning strategies

Crafting flavorful and balanced meals while adhering to a diabetic-friendly approach requires thoughtful recipe ideas and meal planning strategies. By incorporating a variety of nutrient-dense ingredients and considering the glycemic impact of foods, individuals can create delicious and satisfying meals that contribute to stable blood sugar levels. Here are some meal ideas and strategies to inspire a diabetic-friendly culinary journey:

Recipe Ideas:

1. Grilled Salmon with Lemon-Dill Sauce:
   - Marinate salmon fillets in a mixture of lemon juice, olive oil, garlic, and fresh dill.
   - Grill the salmon until it's cooked to perfection.
   - Serve with a side of roasted Brussels sprouts and quinoa for a well-balanced meal.

2. Vegetarian Stir-Fry with Tofu:
   - Stir-fry tofu cubes with a colorful assortment of vegetables such as bell peppers, broccoli, and snap peas.
   - Create a sauce using low-sodium soy sauce, ginger, and garlic.
   - Serve over cauliflower rice or whole-grain brown rice for a satisfying and low-GI option.

3. Mediterranean Chicken Salad:
   - Grilled chicken breast seasoned with Mediterranean herbs, sliced and placed on a bed of mixed greens.
   - Add cherry tomatoes, cucumber, Kalamata olives, and feta cheese.
   - Drizzle with olive oil and balsamic vinegar for a flavorful and nutritious salad.

4. Chickpea and Spinach Curry:
   - Sauté onions, garlic, and ginger in a pot, then add chickpeas, spinach, and diced tomatoes.
   - Season with curry spices like cumin, coriander, and turmeric.
   - Serve over cauliflower rice or quinoa for a fiber-rich and delicious curry.

Meal Planning Strategies:

1. Balanced Plate Approach:
   - Aim for a balanced plate by filling half with non-starchy vegetables, one-quarter with lean protein, and one-quarter with whole grains or legumes.
   - This approach helps control portion sizes and provides a variety of nutrients.

2. Snack Smartly:
   - Plan healthy snacks between meals, such as Greek yogurt with berries, sliced vegetables with hummus, or a handful of nuts.
   - These snacks can help maintain energy levels and prevent overeating during main meals.

3. Prep Ahead for Convenience:
   - Prepare ingredients in advance, such as washing and chopping vegetables, marinating proteins, or cooking grains.
   - Having components ready makes it easier to assemble meals quickly, especially on busy days.

4. Explore Low-GI Foods:
   - Prioritize low-GI foods like sweet potatoes, quinoa, and legumes in meal planning.
   - Experiment with recipes that incorporate these ingredients for sustained energy and blood sugar control.

5. Portion Control with Awareness:
   - Use smaller plates to help control portion sizes naturally.
   - Be mindful of carbohydrate intake by measuring servings and incorporating a variety of colorful vegetables for added nutrients.

6. Hydration Matters:
   - Stay hydrated with water or herbal teas throughout the day.
   - Sometimes, feelings of hunger can be mistaken for dehydration, so maintaining adequate fluid intake is crucial.

By combining these recipe ideas and meal planning strategies, individuals can enjoy a diverse and delicious array of meals while supporting their diabetes management goals. Planning meals mindfully not only contributes to stable blood sugar levels but also enhances the overall enjoyment and satisfaction of the dining experience.

Cooking techniques to preserve nutritional value

Preserving the nutritional value of foods during the cooking process is crucial for maximizing the health benefits of meals. Various cooking techniques can help retain essential nutrients, ensuring that the final dishes are not only delicious but also rich in vitamins, minerals, and other vital components. Here are some cooking techniques that contribute to preserving the nutritional value of foods:

1. Steaming:
   - Steaming is a gentle cooking method that involves exposing food to steam rather than submerging it in water.
   - This technique helps preserve water-soluble vitamins like vitamin C and B-vitamins, which can leach into cooking water.

2. Sautéing:
   - Sautéing quickly cooks food in a small amount of oil over medium to high heat.
   - It's an effective method for retaining the nutritional content of vegetables, as the cooking time is relatively short, minimizing nutrient loss.

3. Grilling:
   - Grilling involves cooking food over an open flame or hot surface.
   - This technique is suitable for lean proteins like chicken or fish and helps maintain their nutritional integrity by allowing excess fats to drip away.

4. Roasting:
  - Roasting involves cooking food in an oven at high temperatures, often with minimal oil.
  - Vegetables, when roasted, can develop a delicious flavor and retain many of their nutrients.

5. Microwaving:
  - Microwaving is a quick and convenient cooking method that uses less water and shorter cooking times.
  - This technique helps preserve the nutritional value of vegetables and is particularly effective for preserving water-soluble vitamins.

6. Blanching:
  - Blanching involves briefly immersing vegetables in boiling water and then quickly cooling them in ice water.
  - This method helps retain color, texture, and nutrients in vegetables while minimizing nutrient loss.

7. Slow Cooking:
  - Slow cooking, such as in a crockpot, allows for long, gentle cooking at low temperatures.
  - This method is suitable for tougher cuts of meat and can help preserve their nutritional content while enhancing flavors.

8. Raw or Lightly Cooked Options:
   - Consuming some fruits and vegetables raw or lightly cooked ensures that they retain their full complement of nutrients.
   - Raw salads, fresh fruit, and vegetable crudités are excellent examples of this approach.

9. Stir-Frying:
   - Stir-frying involves quickly cooking small, uniform pieces of food in a hot pan with minimal oil.
   - This technique retains the texture and nutrients of vegetables, as the cooking time is short.

10. Using Cooking Water:
   - When possible, incorporate cooking water into sauces or soups to capture water-soluble nutrients that may have leached during cooking.

It's essential to note that the choice of cooking technique often depends on the type of food being prepared. Additionally, minimizing overcooking, using minimal amounts of water, and selecting fresh, high-quality ingredients all contribute to preserving the nutritional value of meals. By incorporating these cooking techniques, individuals can strike a balance between creating delicious, well-prepared dishes and retaining the healthful benefits of the ingredients.

Creating satisfying and delicious meals that align with dietary needs

Crafting satisfying and delicious meals that align with specific dietary needs is a creative and rewarding endeavor. This culinary journey involves thoughtful ingredient selection, mindful preparation, and a harmonious balance of flavors to ensure not only nutritional adequacy but also a delightful dining experience.

Begin by embracing a variety of fresh, whole foods that cater to dietary requirements. For those managing diabetes, focus on incorporating low-GI carbohydrates, lean proteins, and healthy fats. This might involve choosing whole grains like quinoa or brown rice, lean protein sources such as poultry or fish, and incorporating heart-healthy fats from avocados, nuts, or olive oil.

Experiment with diverse cooking methods to enhance the natural flavors of ingredients while preserving their nutritional value. Grilling, roasting, or sautéing vegetables and proteins can add depth and complexity to the overall taste. Balancing textures and colors not only contributes to the visual appeal of the meal but also provides a sensory-rich experience.

Herbs and spices become invaluable allies in creating flavorful dishes without relying on excessive salt or sugar. Experiment with aromatic herbs like basil, rosemary, or cilantro, and spices such as cumin, turmeric, or paprika to infuse depth and character into your meals.

Consider incorporating a variety of vegetables to add vibrancy and nutritional density to your dishes. Whether roasted, sautéed, or included in salads, a colorful assortment of vegetables not only contributes essential vitamins and minerals but also elevates the overall palate of the meal.

For those with specific dietary restrictions, explore alternative ingredients and substitutions without compromising taste. Gluten-free grains, plant-based proteins, and dairy alternatives can be seamlessly integrated into recipes to accommodate various dietary needs.

Creating satisfying meals also involves paying attention to portion sizes. Balancing the quantities of proteins, carbohydrates, and fats ensures not only proper nutrition but also a feeling of satiety after meals. Consider using smaller plates to create the illusion of a fuller plate, promoting a mindful approach to portion control.

Lastly, embrace the joy of experimentation in the kitchen. Explore new recipes, cuisines, and cooking techniques to keep meals exciting and diverse. This not only prevents culinary monotony but also opens up a world of possibilities to discover delicious combinations that align with individual dietary requirements.

In essence, the art of creating satisfying and delicious meals that cater to dietary needs is a holistic and dynamic process. It involves a fusion of nutrition science, culinary creativity, and a commitment to well-being. By embracing fresh, nutrient-dense ingredients and thoughtfully preparing meals, individuals can embark on a culinary adventure that not only nourishes the body but also indulges the senses.

Chapter 5: Lifestyle Strategies for Diabetes Management

The role of exercise in blood sugar regulation

Exercise plays a pivotal role in the intricate dance of blood sugar regulation, exerting a profound influence on glucose levels and contributing to overall metabolic health. When individuals engage in physical activity, a cascade of physiological responses occurs, orchestrating a harmonious interplay between muscles, insulin, and energy utilization.

First and foremost, exercise enhances insulin sensitivity, allowing cells to more efficiently absorb glucose from the bloodstream. This effect is particularly significant for individuals with insulin resistance, a common factor in Type 2 diabetes. Through regular physical activity, the body becomes more adept at utilizing insulin, promoting effective glucose uptake by cells and contributing to improved blood sugar control.

Additionally, exercise facilitates muscle contraction, which serves as a natural mechanism for glucose uptake. As muscles contract during physical activity, they utilize glucose for energy. This process occurs independently of insulin, providing an alternative pathway for glucose to enter cells. Regular exercise thus helps to deplete excess glucose from the bloodstream, supporting blood sugar regulation.

Furthermore, engaging in aerobic exercise, such as brisk walking, jogging, or cycling, stimulates the cardiovascular system and increases the demand for oxygen. This heightened demand prompts the body to burn more calories, including stored glucose and fats, to meet the energy requirements of the working muscles. This not only contributes to weight management but also aids in maintaining optimal blood sugar levels.

Resistance training, involving activities like weight lifting or bodyweight exercises, complements aerobic exercise by building lean muscle mass. More muscle mass enhances the body's overall metabolic rate, leading to improved glucose metabolism and increased insulin sensitivity. The combination of aerobic and resistance exercises forms a powerful synergy for blood sugar regulation.

The post-exercise period, commonly known as the "exercise afterburn" or excess post-exercise oxygen consumption (EPOC), represents an additional benefit. Following physical activity, the body continues to burn calories at an elevated rate, promoting further glucose utilization and contributing to sustained blood sugar control even after the workout concludes.

Consistency in incorporating regular exercise into a routine is key to reaping these benefits. Both aerobic and resistance exercises, when integrated into a balanced fitness regimen, become valuable tools for individuals seeking to manage or prevent diabetes. Beyond blood sugar regulation, exercise offers a myriad of additional health advantages, including cardiovascular fitness, weight management, and overall well-being. In essence, the role of exercise in blood sugar regulation extends far beyond the gym or the track, becoming an integral component of a holistic and proactive approach to metabolic health.

Stress management techniques for improved well-being

In the pursuit of improved well-being, effective stress management techniques play a pivotal role in navigating life's challenges and fostering a sense of balance. By incorporating these strategies into daily life, individuals can cultivate resilience, enhance mental health, and promote overall well-being.

1. Mindfulness Meditation:
   - Engage in mindfulness meditation to anchor yourself in the present moment. Focus on your breath, sensations, or a guided meditation to alleviate stress and promote a sense of calm.

2. Deep Breathing Exercises:
   - Practice deep breathing exercises to activate the body's relaxation response. Slow, intentional breaths can reduce physiological stress responses and induce a sense of tranquility.

3. Regular Physical Activity:
   - Incorporate regular exercise into your routine. Physical activity releases endorphins, which act as natural mood elevators, contributing to stress reduction and overall well-being.

4. Time Management:
   - Prioritize tasks and manage time effectively. Break larger tasks into smaller, more manageable steps, and avoid overcommitting. Establishing realistic goals can reduce stress related to time constraints.

5. Positive Affirmations:
   - Foster a positive mindset by practicing affirmations. Encourage self-empowering and optimistic thoughts to counteract negative stress-inducing beliefs.

6. Social Connections:
   - Cultivate strong social connections. Spending time with supportive friends and family provides emotional support and a sense of belonging, which can buffer against stress.

7. Relaxation Techniques:
   - Explore various relaxation techniques, such as progressive muscle relaxation or guided imagery. These methods can help release muscle tension and promote a state of relaxation.

8. Adequate Sleep:
   - Prioritize quality sleep. Establish a consistent sleep routine, create a comfortable sleep environment, and ensure sufficient rest, as sleep

profoundly influences emotional resilience and stress management.

9. Healthy Nutrition:
   - Maintain a balanced and nutritious diet. Proper nutrition supports physical and mental well-being, influencing mood and energy levels, which are key components of stress management.

10. Journaling:
   - Practice journaling as a means of self-reflection. Write down your thoughts, emotions, and experiences to gain insights into sources of stress and identify positive coping strategies.

11. Set Realistic Expectations:
   - Establish realistic expectations for yourself. Recognize that perfection is unattainable, and embrace a mindset that values progress over perfection.

12. Hobbies and Leisure Activities:
   - Engage in hobbies and activities that bring joy and relaxation. Whether it's reading, painting, or spending time in nature, dedicating time to activities you enjoy enhances overall well-being.

13. Professional Support:

- Seek professional support if needed.
Therapists, counselors, or support groups provide
valuable resources for managing stress and
enhancing mental health.

Integrating these stress management techniques
into daily life fosters resilience, promotes
emotional well-being, and equips individuals with
the tools to navigate life's challenges more
effectively. By cultivating a holistic approach to
stress management, individuals can enhance their
overall quality of life and build a foundation for
sustained well-being.

Establishing healthy sleep patterns and their impact on diabetes

Establishing healthy sleep patterns is integral not
only for overall well-being but also for managing
diabetes effectively. The relationship between
sleep and diabetes is intricate, with sleep patterns
influencing various aspects of metabolic health,
insulin sensitivity, and glucose regulation.

Consistent and sufficient sleep duration is crucial for maintaining optimal metabolic function. Inadequate sleep has been associated with insulin resistance, where cells become less responsive to insulin, leading to elevated blood sugar levels. By prioritizing regular sleep patterns and aiming for the recommended 7-9 hours of sleep per night, individuals can support their body's ability to regulate blood glucose levels more effectively.

Furthermore, the circadian rhythm, the body's internal clock, plays a vital role in metabolic processes. Disruptions to the circadian rhythm, often caused by irregular sleep patterns or shift work, can adversely affect glucose metabolism. Establishing a consistent sleep-wake cycle helps synchronize the circadian rhythm, promoting more efficient metabolic function and supporting diabetes management.

Sleep quality is equally important as duration. Conditions like sleep apnea, characterized by interrupted breathing during sleep, are more prevalent in individuals with diabetes. Addressing sleep disorders and ensuring restorative sleep enhances overall health and may contribute to better blood sugar control.

Proper sleep positively influences appetite regulation and weight management, factors intimately linked to diabetes. Sleep deprivation can lead to increased hunger and cravings, particularly for high-calorie, carbohydrate-rich foods. Establishing healthy sleep patterns supports a balanced appetite, making it easier to adhere to a nutritious diet and manage weight effectively.

Moreover, adequate sleep is associated with improved stress management and mental well-being. Chronic stress can contribute to insulin resistance and exacerbate diabetes symptoms. By prioritizing healthy sleep patterns, individuals can enhance their resilience to stressors, fostering a positive impact on both mental and metabolic health.

In summary, healthy sleep patterns play a multifaceted role in diabetes management. By focusing on consistent and sufficient sleep duration, maintaining a regular sleep-wake cycle, and addressing sleep quality, individuals can positively influence insulin sensitivity, glucose regulation, appetite control, and overall well-being. Recognizing the interconnectedness of sleep and diabetes underscores the importance of a holistic approach to health that encompasses lifestyle factors, including sleep, in the pursuit of optimal diabetes management and overall wellness.

Chapter 6: Crafting Your Fitness Routine

Tailoring exercise plans to individual needs

Tailoring exercise plans to individual needs is a cornerstone of effective and sustainable fitness regimens. Recognizing that each person is unique in terms of fitness levels, health conditions, preferences, and goals, a personalized approach ensures that exercise routines are not only enjoyable but also cater to individual capabilities and aspirations.

Assessing Fitness Levels:
   Understanding an individual's current fitness levels is the first step in crafting a tailored exercise plan. This assessment may involve evaluating cardiovascular fitness, muscular strength, flexibility, and other relevant parameters. By establishing a baseline, fitness professionals or individuals themselves can design a program that aligns with their current capabilities.

Considering Health Conditions:
  Individuals often have varying health considerations, such as chronic conditions or previous injuries. Tailoring an exercise plan involves taking these factors into account to ensure that the chosen activities do not exacerbate existing issues. This may involve selecting low-impact exercises, modifying movements, or incorporating specific exercises to address particular health needs.

Setting Realistic Goals:
  Personalized exercise plans are built on realistic and achievable goals. Understanding an individual's objectives—whether it's weight management, improved cardiovascular health, muscle toning, or overall well-being—allows for the customization of exercises that directly contribute to these aspirations. Realistic goals increase motivation and adherence to the exercise routine.

Incorporating Variety and Enjoyment:
  A key aspect of tailoring exercise plans is incorporating activities that individuals enjoy. Whether it's dancing, hiking, swimming, or weightlifting, choosing exercises that align with personal preferences increases the likelihood of long-term commitment. Variety not only keeps

workouts interesting but also ensures a balanced approach to fitness.

Adapting to Preferences and Lifestyle:
  Consideration of lifestyle factors is crucial in tailoring exercise plans. Understanding time constraints, daily schedules, and preferred workout environments allows for the creation of a plan that is realistic and feasible. This adaptability ensures that individuals can seamlessly integrate exercise into their lives without feeling overwhelmed.

Gradual Progression:
  Tailored exercise plans account for the principle of gradual progression. Starting with manageable intensity and gradually increasing the challenge helps prevent injury, allows the body to adapt, and promotes consistent improvement. This approach is particularly important for individuals new to exercise or those returning after a hiatus.

Incorporating Functional Training:
  Addressing functional movements relevant to an individual's daily activities enhances the practicality of an exercise plan. Functional training ensures that exercises translate to improved performance in everyday tasks, contributing not

only to fitness but also to enhanced overall functionality.

Regular Monitoring and Adjustments:
   Personalized exercise plans are dynamic and require periodic assessment. Regular monitoring of progress allows for adjustments based on individual responses to the program. This iterative process ensures that the exercise plan evolves to meet changing needs and goals over time.

In essence, tailoring exercise plans to individual needs involves a holistic understanding of each person's unique characteristics, preferences, and objectives. This personalized approach not only enhances the effectiveness of the exercise routine but also promotes sustained engagement and, ultimately, long-term fitness success.

Workout Routine

A well-rounded workout routine for individuals with diabetes should encompass both aerobic exercises and strength training, promoting cardiovascular health, insulin sensitivity, and overall well-being. Here's a brief workout routine that combines these elements:

Warm-Up:
  - Start with 5-10 minutes of light aerobic activity, such as brisk walking or jogging in place, to increase blood flow and prepare muscles for exercise.
  - Include dynamic stretches to gently stretch major muscle groups.

Aerobic Exercise (Cardiovascular):
  - Engage in 30 minutes of moderate-intensity aerobic exercise most days of the week.
  - Options include brisk walking, cycling, swimming, dancing, or low-impact aerobics.
  - Modify intensity based on individual fitness levels, aiming for a perceived exertion level that is challenging but sustainable.

Strength Training:
  - Incorporate strength training exercises at least two days a week.
  - Focus on major muscle groups, including legs, arms, chest, back, and core.
  - Use bodyweight exercises like squats, lunges, push-ups, and planks, or incorporate resistance training with resistance bands or light weights.

Flexibility and Balance:
  - Dedicate 5-10 minutes to flexibility exercises and balance training.

   - Include stretches for major muscle groups, holding each stretch for 15-30 seconds.
   - Practice balance exercises, such as single-leg stands or heel-to-toe walking.

Cool Down:
   - Finish with 5-10 minutes of light aerobic activity to gradually lower heart rate.
   - Include static stretches to further improve flexibility and reduce muscle tension.

Guidelines:
   - Check blood sugar levels before and after exercise, especially if using insulin or certain medications that can affect blood sugar.
   - Stay hydrated throughout the workout.
   - Listen to your body and modify exercises as needed.
   - If you have any existing health conditions, consult with a healthcare professional before starting a new exercise routine.

Balancing aerobic and strength training for optimal results

Achieving optimal fitness results involves striking a harmonious balance between aerobic exercise and strength training. This dual approach not only enhances overall physical fitness but also provides a well-rounded strategy for health and wellness.

Aerobic exercise, such as brisk walking, running, or cycling, elevates the heart rate and improves cardiovascular health. It enhances endurance, burns calories, and contributes to weight management. Regular aerobic activity also has profound benefits for blood sugar control, particularly beneficial for individuals managing diabetes. The rhythmic nature of aerobic exercises engages large muscle groups, promoting efficient oxygen utilization and overall cardiovascular efficiency.

Complementing aerobic exercise with strength training adds a crucial dimension to fitness. Strength training, which involves resistance exercises like weightlifting or bodyweight exercises, enhances muscular strength, tone, and endurance. Building lean muscle mass is not only aesthetically beneficial but also contributes to a higher metabolic rate, aiding in weight management and overall energy expenditure.

Balancing these two components creates a synergistic effect. Aerobic exercise serves as a foundation for cardiovascular health and weight management, while strength training adds structural integrity to the body, supporting joint health and preventing muscle imbalances. The combination is particularly effective in enhancing functional fitness, allowing individuals to perform daily activities with greater ease and reducing the risk of injuries.

Moreover, this dual approach positively influences metabolism. While aerobic exercise burns calories during the activity, strength training contributes to an "afterburn" effect, where the body continues to burn calories at an elevated rate after the workout. This combination supports both weight loss and muscle maintenance or growth.

Importantly, the balance between aerobic and strength training is adaptable to individual goals. For those aiming primarily for cardiovascular fitness, a higher emphasis on aerobic exercise may be suitable. Conversely, individuals focusing on building muscle or improving strength may allocate more time to strength training. The key is to recognize the complementary nature of these exercise modalities and integrate them in a way that aligns with individual preferences, fitness levels, and long-term goals.

In essence, the optimal results in fitness are found in the synergy of aerobic exercise and strength training. This balanced approach not only promotes physical health but also contributes to mental well-being, offering a holistic and sustainable path to achieving and maintaining overall fitness.

Overcoming common barriers to staying active

Staying active is a key component of a healthy lifestyle, but various barriers can hinder individuals from maintaining regular physical activity. Overcoming these common obstacles requires a proactive and adaptable approach that addresses both physical and psychological challenges.

One prevalent barrier is a lack of time. Busy schedules and competing priorities can make carving out time for exercise seem challenging. To overcome this, individuals can schedule physical activity as they would any other important commitment. Incorporating shorter, more frequent bouts of exercise throughout the day can also be an effective strategy, making it more achievable within tight schedules.

Another common barrier is the perception that exercise has to be strenuous or time-consuming. Adopting a more flexible mindset towards physical activity can help. Recognizing that even short, moderate-intensity activities contribute to overall health can make it easier to incorporate movement into daily life. Finding enjoyable activities further motivates consistent participation.

Environmental factors, such as unfavorable weather or limited access to exercise facilities, can also impede regular activity. Adapting to these challenges might involve exploring indoor workout options, utilizing home-based exercises, or identifying alternative outdoor activities that align with the current conditions. Flexibility in choosing activities based on the environment enhances the likelihood of continued engagement.

Lack of motivation or boredom is another barrier to staying active. Incorporating variety into workouts, trying new activities, or exercising with a friend or group can inject enthusiasm into the routine. Setting specific, achievable goals and celebrating milestones creates a sense of accomplishment, reinforcing the motivation to stay active.

Physical limitations or health concerns may present significant barriers. It's crucial to consult with healthcare professionals to design a safe and suitable exercise plan. Tailoring activities to individual abilities, considering low-impact options, and focusing on activities that bring joy can help overcome these barriers while promoting overall well-being.

Social factors, such as a lack of social support or feeling self-conscious during exercise, can also hinder physical activity. Engaging in group activities, joining fitness classes, or seeking support from friends and family create a positive social environment. Embracing the mindset that everyone has different fitness levels and goals can alleviate self-consciousness and enhance the enjoyment of physical activity.

Overcoming common barriers to staying active involves a combination of planning, flexibility, and a positive mindset. By addressing time constraints, redefining the perception of exercise, adapting to environmental factors, finding motivation, considering individual health needs, and fostering social connections, individuals can build habits that promote regular physical activity and contribute to a healthier and more active lifestyle.

Chapter 7: Stress Reduction Techniques

Mindfulness and meditation practices for stress relief

Mindfulness and meditation practices offer powerful tools for stress relief, promoting a sense of calm and resilience in the face of life's challenges. By cultivating awareness and being present in the moment, individuals can effectively manage stress and enhance overall well-being.

Mindfulness Meditation:
   Engage in mindfulness meditation to ground yourself in the present moment. Find a quiet space, sit comfortably, and focus your attention on your breath. Allow thoughts to come and go without judgment, gently bringing your focus back to the breath. Mindfulness meditation can be practiced for as little as a few minutes or extended for longer sessions.

Body Scan Meditation:
   Practice a body scan meditation to promote relaxation and release physical tension. Close your

eyes and bring awareness to different parts of your body, starting from your toes and gradually moving up to the top of your head. Notice any sensations or areas of tension, and consciously release any tightness or discomfort as you breathe.

Loving-Kindness Meditation:
   Engage in loving-kindness meditation to cultivate feelings of compassion and connection. Begin by focusing on sending well-wishes to yourself, then extend these wishes to loved ones, acquaintances, and even those with whom you may have challenges. This practice fosters a sense of goodwill and can counteract stress by promoting positive emotions.

Guided Meditation:
   Utilize guided meditations, which are led by an instructor or available through various apps and online platforms. These sessions often provide a structured approach to relaxation, guiding you through visualizations, breathing exercises, and mindfulness techniques. Guided meditations can be particularly helpful for beginners.

Mindful Breathing Exercises:
   Incorporate mindful breathing exercises into your daily routine. Whether it's deep

diaphragmatic breathing, box breathing, or simply paying attention to each inhale and exhale, conscious breathing can quickly shift your focus away from stressors and induce a sense of calm.

Mindful Walking:
   Practice mindful walking to combine physical activity with mindfulness. Pay attention to each step, the sensation of your feet making contact with the ground, and your breath as you walk. This simple activity can be done anywhere, providing a refreshing break and an opportunity to center yourself.

Mindful Eating:
   Bring mindfulness to your meals by savoring each bite, paying attention to flavors, textures, and smells. Eating mindfully can create a more enjoyable dining experience and help break the cycle of stress-related eating.

Daily Mindfulness Practices:
   Infuse mindfulness into daily activities such as washing dishes, commuting, or even waiting in line. By bringing full attention to these routine moments, you can transform them into opportunities for relaxation and stress reduction.

Regular practice of mindfulness and meditation develops a heightened awareness that extends beyond the meditation sessions, fostering a sense of presence and resilience in everyday life. As you integrate these practices into your routine, you may find that they become valuable tools for navigating stress, promoting emotional well-being, and cultivating a more mindful approach to life's experiences.

Building resilience to navigate daily challenges

Building resilience is a dynamic process that empowers individuals to navigate daily challenges with strength, adaptability, and a positive mindset. Resilience involves cultivating the ability to bounce back from setbacks, learn from experiences, and thrive despite adversity.

One fundamental aspect of building resilience is developing a healthy mindset. This entails reframing negative thoughts into more positive and constructive perspectives. Rather than viewing challenges as insurmountable obstacles, individuals with resilience see them as opportunities for growth and learning. Embracing a mindset that acknowledges setbacks as temporary and solvable contributes significantly to building emotional strength.

Cultivating self-awareness is another key component of resilience. This involves understanding one's emotions, reactions, and coping mechanisms. By recognizing personal strengths and areas for improvement, individuals can better navigate challenges and make informed choices. Regular self-reflection fosters a deeper understanding of one's values, priorities, and goals, laying the foundation for resilient responses to adversity.

Effective stress management plays a vital role in building resilience. Adopting healthy coping strategies, such as mindfulness, meditation, or physical exercise, helps regulate emotions and reduce the impact of stressors. By incorporating these practices into daily life, individuals create a robust support system for their mental and emotional well-being, enhancing their ability to face challenges with composure.

Establishing and maintaining a strong social support network is another resilience-building strategy. Meaningful connections with friends, family, or community provide emotional support during tough times. Sharing experiences, seeking advice, or simply knowing that there is a network of support fosters a sense of belonging and reinforces an individual's capacity to overcome difficulties.

Flexibility and adaptability are crucial elements of resilience. Life is inherently unpredictable, and being able to adapt to change is a valuable skill. Resilient individuals approach challenges with a willingness to adjust their goals or plans as needed. This adaptive mindset allows for a more fluid response to unforeseen circumstances, reducing the impact of stressors on overall well-being.

Setting realistic goals and breaking them into manageable steps is a practical approach to building resilience. By achieving small victories, individuals build confidence in their ability to overcome challenges. This incremental progress contributes to a sense of accomplishment and reinforces the belief that one can handle adversity effectively.

Moreover, fostering a positive and optimistic outlook contributes significantly to resilience. Emphasizing positive aspects of situations, no matter how small, helps shift focus away from negativity. This positive orientation not only influences emotional well-being but also enhances problem-solving skills and the ability to find solutions amid challenges.

In essence, building resilience is an ongoing and intentional process that involves developing a positive mindset, cultivating self-awareness, managing stress effectively, fostering social connections, embracing adaptability, setting realistic goals, and maintaining a positive outlook. By integrating these elements into daily life, individuals empower themselves to navigate challenges with resilience, ultimately leading to greater overall well-being and a more fulfilling life journey.

Creating a supportive environment for emotional well-being

Creating a supportive environment for emotional well-being involves fostering surroundings that promote mental health, resilience, and a sense of belonging. This comprehensive approach encompasses various aspects of life and influences, working synergistically to contribute to overall emotional well-being.

Positive Social Connections:
   Building and maintaining positive social connections is foundational. A supportive environment is one where individuals can openly share their thoughts and feelings without judgment. Cultivating healthy relationships, whether with family, friends, or a broader community, provides a crucial foundation for emotional support.

Open Communication:
   Encouraging open and honest communication within relationships contributes to a supportive emotional environment. Creating a space where individuals feel heard, validated, and understood fosters a sense of security and reinforces the notion that emotions are acknowledged and valued.

Empathy and Understanding:

Infusing empathy into interactions is essential. A supportive environment acknowledges the diverse range of emotions individuals may experience and responds with empathy and understanding. This creates a culture that embraces emotional expression and validates the complexity of human feelings.

Promoting Work-Life Balance:
Striking a healthy balance between work and personal life is vital. A supportive environment recognizes the importance of downtime, relaxation, and self-care. This approach not only reduces stress but also reinforces the idea that well-being extends beyond professional responsibilities.

Physical Well-Being:
The connection between physical health and emotional well-being is undeniable. A supportive environment promotes healthy lifestyle choices, including regular exercise, nutritious eating, and sufficient sleep. These elements contribute to both physical and mental resilience.

Encouraging Self-Reflection:
A supportive environment encourages self-reflection. Providing opportunities for individuals to explore their thoughts and emotions, perhaps

through journaling or mindfulness practices, fosters self-awareness. This introspective aspect contributes to personal growth and emotional resilience.

Flexible and Inclusive Policies:
In workplaces or communities, implementing flexible and inclusive policies supports emotional well-being. This may involve accommodating diverse needs, recognizing the importance of mental health days, or fostering a culture that values the unique contributions of each individual.

Reducing Stigma:
Creating an environment that actively works to reduce the stigma surrounding mental health is crucial. This involves open discussions, education, and initiatives that promote understanding and empathy towards individuals facing mental health challenges.

Promoting a Positive Culture:
Cultivating a positive culture within a family, workplace, or community reinforces emotional well-being. This involves celebrating achievements, expressing gratitude, and focusing on strengths. A positive culture contributes to a sense of optimism and shared purpose.

Access to Resources and Support:
   A supportive environment ensures access to resources and support services for those in need. This may include mental health resources, counseling services, or community support groups. Knowing that help is available reinforces a sense of security and encourages individuals to seek assistance when required.

In essence, creating a supportive environment for emotional well-being involves weaving together various threads of positive social connections, open communication, empathy, work-life balance, physical well-being, self-reflection, flexible policies, stigma reduction, positive culture, and access to resources. This holistic approach recognizes the interconnectedness of these elements, working collectively to nurture emotional resilience and foster a thriving environment for individuals to navigate life's challenges.

Chapter 8: The Power of Quality Sleep

Understanding the link between sleep and blood sugar control

The intricate link between sleep and blood sugar control is a dynamic interplay that significantly influences overall metabolic health. This relationship is multifaceted, encompassing hormonal regulation, glucose metabolism, and the delicate balance of various physiological processes.

At the core of this connection lies the impact of sleep duration and quality on insulin sensitivity. Insulin, a hormone produced by the pancreas, plays a pivotal role in facilitating the uptake of glucose by cells for energy. Inadequate or poor-quality sleep disrupts this delicate dance, leading to reduced insulin sensitivity. As a result, cells become less responsive to insulin, and glucose absorption is compromised, ultimately contributing to elevated blood sugar levels.

Moreover, sleep deprivation can disturb the balance of other key hormones involved in glucose regulation. Ghrelin, known as the hunger hormone, tends to increase with insufficient sleep, potentially leading to elevated appetite and a preference for high-calorie, carbohydrate-rich foods. Conversely, leptin, the hormone responsible for signaling satiety, decreases, further influencing dietary choices and potentially contributing to weight gain.

The circadian rhythm, the body's internal clock that regulates various physiological processes over a 24-hour cycle, also plays a crucial role in this intricate relationship. Disruptions to the circadian rhythm, such as irregular sleep patterns or shift work, can lead to misalignment between the body's natural cycles and external cues. This misalignment can impact the timing of insulin release and glucose metabolism, contributing to challenges in blood sugar control.

Furthermore, the restorative aspect of sleep contributes to overall stress reduction. Chronic stress can trigger the release of cortisol, a hormone that influences blood sugar levels. Inadequate sleep, coupled with heightened stress, creates a physiological environment that may contribute to fluctuations in blood sugar.

Understanding the link between sleep and blood sugar control emphasizes the importance of prioritizing healthy sleep habits as a fundamental component of diabetes management and overall well-being. Consistent, sufficient sleep supports optimal insulin sensitivity, hormonal balance, and circadian rhythm alignment, all crucial factors for effective blood sugar regulation.

In practical terms, fostering good sleep hygiene involves maintaining a regular sleep schedule, creating a comfortable sleep environment, and adopting relaxation practices before bedtime. By recognizing the profound impact of sleep on metabolic health, individuals can take proactive steps to prioritize sleep as a cornerstone of their diabetes management strategy and overall health promotion.

Establishing a sleep routine for better diabetes management

Establishing a consistent sleep routine is a foundational element in the comprehensive approach to better diabetes management. The significance of a well-structured sleep routine extends beyond mere rest; it directly influences factors such as insulin sensitivity, glucose regulation, and overall metabolic health.

The cornerstone of an effective sleep routine is maintaining a consistent sleep schedule. Going to bed and waking up at the same time each day, even on weekends, helps regulate the body's internal clock, reinforcing the circadian rhythm. This consistency optimizes the timing of various physiological processes, including insulin release, contributing to improved blood sugar control.

Creating a conducive sleep environment is equally crucial. The bedroom should be cool, dark, and quiet, promoting a comfortable atmosphere for restorative sleep. Eliminating electronic devices at least an hour before bedtime minimizes exposure to blue light, which can interfere with the production of the sleep-inducing hormone melatonin.

Engaging in a calming pre-sleep routine signals to the body that it's time to wind down. Activities such as reading a book, practicing relaxation techniques, or taking a warm bath can help transition from the busyness of the day to a more relaxed state conducive to sleep. These rituals contribute to stress reduction, an important factor in supporting overall diabetes management.

Being mindful of dietary choices, especially in the evening, plays a role in optimizing sleep quality. Consuming heavy or high-sugar meals close to bedtime can disrupt sleep patterns and influence blood sugar levels. Establishing a routine of balanced, nutritious meals throughout the day and avoiding stimulants like caffeine in the evening contributes to both better sleep and improved metabolic health.

Regular physical activity is a valuable component of diabetes management, and it also contributes to better sleep. Incorporating exercise into the daily routine, preferably earlier in the day, can enhance sleep quality. However, vigorous exercise close to bedtime may have stimulating effects, so timing is essential for maximizing its benefits on both sleep and diabetes.

Minimizing stressors and creating a sense of relaxation before bedtime further supports a healthy sleep routine. Mindfulness practices, such as meditation or deep-breathing exercises, can be effective tools for calming the mind and reducing stress levels. Managing stress is particularly important for individuals with diabetes, as chronic stress can impact blood sugar control.

In essence, establishing a sleep routine for better diabetes management involves the integration of consistent sleep schedules, a conducive sleep environment, pre-sleep relaxation rituals, mindful dietary choices, regular physical activity, and stress management practices. By prioritizing a comprehensive approach to sleep hygiene, individuals with diabetes can harness the benefits of quality sleep to positively impact their metabolic health and overall well-being.

Tips for addressing common sleep disturbances

Addressing common sleep disturbances involves adopting strategies that promote better sleep hygiene and addressing factors that may contribute to disruptions in sleep patterns. Here are practical tips to help improve sleep quality:

1. Maintain a Consistent Sleep Schedule:
   Go to bed and wake up at the same time every day, even on weekends. Consistency reinforces the body's internal clock, promoting better sleep-wake cycles.

2. Create a Relaxing Bedtime Routine:
   Establish a calming pre-sleep routine to signal to your body that it's time to wind down. Engage in activities such as reading, gentle stretching, or practicing relaxation techniques before bedtime.

3. Optimize Sleep Environment:
   Ensure your bedroom is conducive to sleep. Keep the room cool, dark, and quiet. Invest in a comfortable mattress and pillows to enhance overall sleep comfort.

4. Limit Exposure to Screens Before Bed:
   Minimize exposure to electronic devices at least an hour before bedtime. The blue light emitted from screens can interfere with the production of the sleep-inducing hormone melatonin.

5. Be Mindful of Diet and Hydration:
   Avoid heavy meals, caffeine, and excessive liquids close to bedtime. Opt for a light snack if hungry. These choices can impact digestion and

reduce the likelihood of disruptions during the night.

6. Regular Physical Activity:
   Engage in regular physical activity, but try to finish intense workouts a few hours before bedtime. Regular exercise can promote better sleep, but timing is essential to avoid stimulating effects close to bedtime.

7. Manage Stress and Anxiety:
   Practice stress-reducing techniques such as meditation, deep breathing, or progressive muscle relaxation. Managing stress and anxiety can significantly improve sleep quality.

8. Evaluate and Improve Sleep Environment:
   Assess your bedroom for potential sleep disturbances. Address issues such as noise, light, or uncomfortable bedding to create an optimal sleep environment.

9. Limit Naps During the Day:
   If you need to nap during the day, keep it short (20-30 minutes) and avoid napping too close to bedtime. Long or late-afternoon naps can interfere with nighttime sleep.

10. Consider Cognitive Behavioral Therapy for Insomnia (CBT-I):
   CBT-I is a structured program that helps address thoughts and behaviors that contribute to insomnia. Consult with a healthcare professional to explore this therapeutic approach.

11. Limit Stimulants Before Bed:
   Minimize the consumption of stimulants like caffeine and nicotine in the hours leading up to bedtime. These substances can interfere with falling asleep and disrupt sleep quality.

12. Seek Professional Help if Needed:
   If sleep disturbances persist, consult with a healthcare professional. Chronic sleep issues may require further evaluation, and a healthcare provider can offer personalized advice or recommend additional interventions.

By incorporating these tips into your routine and making adjustments as needed, you can address common sleep disturbances and foster healthier sleep habits. Consistency and a holistic approach to sleep hygiene contribute to better overall sleep quality and promote well-being.

Chapter 9: Integrating Lifestyle Changes

Developing a personalized diabetes management plan

Developing a personalized diabetes management plan involves tailoring strategies to individual needs, considering factors such as lifestyle, preferences, health conditions, and overall well-being. This comprehensive approach encompasses various aspects to effectively manage blood sugar levels and promote overall health.

1. Consult with Healthcare Professionals:
   Begin by consulting with a healthcare team, including a primary care physician, endocrinologist, and/or diabetes educator. These professionals can provide a thorough assessment of your health, offer personalized advice, and guide the development of a tailored diabetes management plan.

2. Establish Blood Sugar Targets:
   Work with your healthcare team to set specific blood sugar targets tailored to your individual needs and health goals. These targets will serve as a benchmark for monitoring and adjusting your diabetes management plan.

3. Develop a Nutritious Eating Plan:
   Collaborate with a registered dietitian or nutritionist to create a personalized eating plan. Consider factors such as carbohydrate intake, portion control, and meal timing. Emphasize a balanced diet rich in fruits, vegetables, lean proteins, and whole grains.

4. Incorporate Regular Physical Activity:
   Design an exercise routine that aligns with your fitness level, preferences, and health conditions. This may include aerobic exercises, strength training, and flexibility exercises. Regular physical activity can enhance insulin sensitivity and contribute to overall well-being.

5. Medication Management:
   If prescribed medication, adhere to the recommended dosage and schedule. Discuss any concerns or side effects with your healthcare provider. Adjustments to medication may be

necessary based on blood sugar monitoring and overall health.

6. Monitor Blood Sugar Levels:
   Establish a routine for monitoring blood sugar levels, and work with your healthcare team to interpret and respond to the results. Regular monitoring provides valuable insights into the effectiveness of your diabetes management plan and helps identify trends.

7. Stress Management:
   Integrate stress management techniques into your routine, such as mindfulness, deep breathing, or yoga. Chronic stress can impact blood sugar levels, and incorporating stress-reducing practices contributes to overall well-being.

8. Adequate Sleep:
   Prioritize quality sleep by establishing a consistent sleep routine. Aim for 7-9 hours of sleep per night, as sleep plays a crucial role in blood sugar control and overall health.

9. Regular Healthcare Check-ups:
   Schedule regular check-ups with your healthcare team to assess overall health, review blood test

results, and make adjustments to your diabetes management plan as needed.

10. Diabetes Education and Support:
   Stay informed about diabetes through educational resources and support groups. Understanding your condition empowers you to make informed decisions about your health. Seek support from friends, family, or diabetes support communities.

11. Hydration:
   Ensure proper hydration by drinking an adequate amount of water throughout the day. Staying hydrated supports various bodily functions and can contribute to overall health.

12. Periodic Plan Review:
   Regularly review and adjust your diabetes management plan in collaboration with your healthcare team. Lifestyle changes, health conditions, or other factors may necessitate modifications to optimize your plan over time.

A personalized diabetes management plan is an evolving framework that adapts to your changing needs and circumstances. Regular communication with healthcare professionals, self-monitoring, and a commitment to a healthy lifestyle form the foundation for effective diabetes management tailored to your unique requirements.

Setting realistic goals for sustainable lifestyle changes

Establishing realistic goals for sustainable lifestyle changes involves a thoughtful and comprehensive approach that considers individual capabilities, preferences, and long-term aspirations. This process revolves around creating a framework that not only motivates initial changes but also sets the stage for continuous progress and lasting habits.

Understanding Individual Capabilities:
Begin by recognizing your current capabilities, taking into account physical health, fitness levels, and any potential limitations. Assessing your starting point provides a realistic foundation for setting achievable goals that align with your unique circumstances.

Identifying Personal Motivations:

Explore the reasons behind your desire for lifestyle changes. Whether it's improving overall health, managing a specific condition, or enhancing well-being, understanding your motivations helps shape goals that resonate personally. Aligning goals with intrinsic motivations enhances commitment and long-term adherence.

Gradual Progression Over Drastic Changes:
Rather than opting for drastic and unsustainable changes, prioritize gradual progression. Break down larger objectives into smaller, manageable steps. This incremental approach not only makes goals more achievable but also fosters a sense of accomplishment, motivating you to sustain your efforts.

Focusing on Behavioral Changes:
Shift the focus from outcome-based goals to behavioral changes. Instead of solely targeting a specific weight or blood sugar level, concentrate on establishing habits that contribute to those outcomes. For instance, set goals related to regular exercise, balanced nutrition, or stress management, emphasizing the process over immediate results.

Incorporating Flexibility:

Recognize that life is dynamic, and unforeseen circumstances may arise. Build flexibility into your goals to accommodate fluctuations in schedules, priorities, or unexpected challenges. This adaptability ensures that setbacks are viewed as temporary obstacles rather than insurmountable barriers.

Setting Specific, Measurable, Attainable, Relevant, and Time-bound (SMART) Goals:
Utilize the SMART criteria to structure your goals. Ensure they are Specific (clear and concise), Measurable (quantifiable), Attainable (realistic), Relevant (aligned with your values and aspirations), and Time-bound (with a set timeframe). This framework provides clarity and accountability in goal-setting.

Celebrating Milestones Along the Journey:
Acknowledge and celebrate small victories and milestones throughout your journey. Recognizing achievements, no matter how modest, reinforces positive behaviors and fosters a sense of motivation. Regularly reflecting on progress helps maintain momentum and enthusiasm for sustainable changes.

Incorporating Enjoyable Activities:

Integrate activities and choices that bring joy and satisfaction. Whether it's finding pleasure in certain exercises, exploring new recipes, or engaging in hobbies that promote well-being, incorporating enjoyment into your lifestyle changes makes them more sustainable and fulfilling.

Seeking Support and Accountability:
Share your goals with friends, family, or a support network. Having a support system provides encouragement and accountability. Regular check-ins or collaborating with others who share similar objectives can enhance motivation and commitment.

Periodic Reflection and Adjustment:
Regularly reflect on your goals, assessing what is working well and identifying areas for adjustment. A willingness to adapt your goals based on changing circumstances or insights gained along the way contributes to the sustainability of your lifestyle changes.

By weaving these principles into the fabric of your goal-setting process, you create a foundation for sustainable lifestyle changes. This approach not only fosters immediate progress but also lays the groundwork for lasting habits that contribute to improved overall well-being and a healthier, more fulfilling life.

Monitoring progress and adapting strategies as needed

Monitoring progress and adapting strategies as needed is a fundamental aspect of any journey toward sustainable lifestyle changes. As you embark on this transformative path, the ability to consistently assess your efforts, recognize achievements, and make informed adjustments becomes a dynamic process that fuels ongoing success.

Regularly tracking your progress provides valuable insights into the effectiveness of your chosen strategies. Whether your focus is on fitness, nutrition, stress management, or overall well-being, keeping a watchful eye on how your body responds and how you feel can reveal patterns and trends over time. This self-awareness becomes a compass, guiding you toward areas that require attention and acknowledging aspects where you're making strides.

One key to successful monitoring is establishing measurable benchmarks or milestones. These can be quantitative, such as tracking physical activity levels, dietary choices, or specific health metrics, or qualitative, involving reflections on mood, energy levels, and overall satisfaction. The combination of objective measurements and subjective assessments paints a comprehensive picture of your progress.

Celebrating achievements, no matter how small, plays a crucial role in maintaining motivation and momentum. Recognizing milestones, whether it's achieving a fitness goal, consistently adhering to a balanced nutrition plan, or effectively managing stress, reinforces positive behaviors. This acknowledgment fosters a sense of accomplishment and reinforces your commitment to the journey.

However, the path to sustainable lifestyle changes is rarely a linear trajectory. Setbacks or challenges are natural components of any transformative process. The ability to view setbacks not as failures but as opportunities for learning and adjustment is a key mindset shift. Instead of becoming discouraged, consider setbacks as data points guiding you to refine your strategies or reevaluate your goals.

Adaptability is a powerful ally in the pursuit of sustainable changes. As circumstances evolve, your strategies should be flexible enough to accommodate these changes. Life is dynamic, and what works at one point may need modification later on. Being open to adjusting your goals, routines, or approaches based on new insights or changing circumstances ensures that your efforts remain relevant and effective.

Seeking support from others is a valuable component of progress monitoring. Sharing your journey with friends, family, or a support network provides an external perspective, encouragement, and often, helpful insights. Regular check-ins or collaborating with others who share similar objectives can offer accountability and motivation, making the process more rewarding.

Periodic reflection on your overall well-being, not just specific goals, contributes to a holistic approach. Assess how your lifestyle changes are impacting your mood, energy levels, sleep quality, and general satisfaction with life. These broader reflections offer a more nuanced understanding of your progress and contribute to a more comprehensive sense of well-being.

In essence, monitoring progress and adapting strategies as needed is an ongoing and iterative process. It involves keen self-awareness, measurable benchmarks, celebrating achievements, viewing setbacks as opportunities for learning, embracing adaptability, seeking support, and reflecting on holistic well-being. This dynamic approach not only enhances the likelihood of sustained success but also transforms the journey of lifestyle changes into a continuous and fulfilling process of self-discovery and growth.

Conclusion: Thriving with Diabetes
- Summarizing key takeaways
In summary, the journey towards sustainable lifestyle changes involves a thoughtful and personalized approach. Begin by setting realistic goals that align with your individual capabilities and motivations. Focus on gradual progression, emphasizing behavioral changes rather than immediate outcomes. Utilize the SMART criteria to structure your goals, ensuring they are Specific, Measurable, Attainable, Relevant, and Time-bound.

A crucial aspect of this transformative journey is developing a comprehensive diabetes management plan. Consult with healthcare professionals to establish blood sugar targets, create a nutritious eating plan, and incorporate regular physical activity. Emphasize flexibility, recognizing that adjustments to the plan may be necessary based on evolving circumstances or health conditions.

Create a supportive environment for emotional well-being by fostering positive social connections, encouraging open communication, and promoting work-life balance. Address stress through mindfulness practices and incorporate relaxation techniques into your routine. Reduce stigma surrounding mental health and ensure access to resources and support for emotional well-being.

Prioritize quality sleep by establishing a consistent sleep routine and creating a conducive sleep environment. Recognize the intricate link between sleep and blood sugar control, understanding how sleep influences insulin sensitivity, hormonal regulation, and overall metabolic health.

As you embark on this transformative journey, monitor progress regularly and adapt strategies as needed. Track measurable benchmarks, celebrate achievements, and view setbacks as opportunities for learning and adjustment. Embrace adaptability, seeking support from a network of friends, family, or support groups.

In essence, the key takeaways emphasize a holistic and individualized approach to diabetes management and overall well-being. By integrating these principles into your lifestyle, you can cultivate sustainable habits, navigate challenges effectively, and foster a fulfilling and health-focused life journey.

Empowering individuals to embrace a holistic approach to diabetes care

Empowering individuals to embrace a holistic approach to diabetes care is a transformative endeavor that goes beyond the management of blood sugar levels. This comprehensive approach recognizes the intricate interplay between various aspects of life and aims to foster overall well-being for those living with diabetes.

At the core of this empowerment is the importance of setting realistic and individualized goals. By understanding personal motivations and capabilities, individuals can tailor their diabetes management plans to align with their unique circumstances. Gradual progression, focusing on behavioral changes, and incorporating flexibility into goal-setting contribute to sustained efforts over time.

A cornerstone of holistic diabetes care is the development of a well-rounded diabetes management plan. Collaboration with healthcare professionals is essential to establish blood sugar targets, create balanced nutrition plans, and integrate regular physical activity. The emphasis is not only on achieving specific outcomes but also on cultivating habits that positively impact overall health.

Creating a supportive environment for emotional well-being is integral to holistic care. This involves fostering positive social connections, promoting open communication, and addressing stress through mindfulness practices. By reducing stigma around mental health and ensuring access to resources, individuals can enhance their emotional resilience and well-being.

Recognizing the vital link between sleep and blood sugar control is paramount in this holistic approach. Establishing consistent sleep routines, creating conducive sleep environments, and understanding how sleep influences insulin sensitivity contribute to an overarching strategy for metabolic health.

The journey towards holistic diabetes care involves regular monitoring of progress and adapting strategies as needed. Acknowledging achievements, viewing setbacks as opportunities for learning, and embracing adaptability are integral components of this dynamic process. Seeking support from a network of friends, family, or support groups provides encouragement and reinforces a sense of community in the face of challenges.

In essence, empowering individuals to embrace a holistic approach to diabetes care transcends the conventional focus on blood sugar management. It involves nurturing physical, emotional, and social well-being through personalized goal-setting, collaborative healthcare efforts, and a commitment to continuous self-improvement. By integrating these principles into their lives, individuals can navigate the complexities of diabetes with resilience, fostering a holistic and fulfilling approach to overall health and wellness.

Encouraging lifelong habits for improved health and well-being.

Encouraging lifelong habits for improved health and well-being is a visionary commitment that recognizes the enduring impact of sustained positive choices on an individual's overall quality of life. This endeavor goes beyond short-term fixes and seeks to instill habits that become integral parts of daily routines, contributing to long-lasting vitality and wellness.

Central to this encouragement is the cultivation of habits that align with an individual's values, preferences, and aspirations. By tailoring health practices to resonate with personal motivations, individuals are more likely to embrace and maintain these habits over the course of their lives. The emphasis is on creating a seamless integration of health-conscious choices into the fabric of one's lifestyle.

A crucial aspect of fostering lifelong habits is the recognition that change is a gradual process. Rather than focusing on rapid transformations, the approach is to introduce adjustments gradually, allowing individuals to adapt and internalize new behaviors. This incremental strategy not only enhances the sustainability of these habits but also promotes a sense of achievement and empowerment.

Holistic well-being is at the forefront of encouraging lifelong habits. This involves addressing various dimensions of health, including physical, emotional, social, and mental aspects. By recognizing the interconnectedness of these elements, individuals can develop a comprehensive set of habits that contribute to a balanced and fulfilling life.

Nutrition plays a pivotal role in this holistic approach. Encouraging habits related to mindful eating, balanced nutrition, and portion control contributes not only to physical health but also to the cultivation of a positive relationship with food. This extends beyond short-term dietary restrictions to a sustainable and enjoyable approach to nourishment.

Regular physical activity is another cornerstone of lifelong habits for improved well-being. Rather than viewing exercise as a temporary obligation, the encouragement is to find activities that bring joy and can be seamlessly integrated into daily life. This shift in perspective transforms exercise from a chore into a rewarding and sustainable lifestyle habit.

Mindfulness practices, stress management techniques, and adequate sleep are integral components of the holistic approach. Encouraging habits related to these aspects fosters emotional resilience, mental clarity, and overall psychological well-being. By incorporating these practices, individuals create a foundation for enduring health and vitality.

The encouragement of lifelong habits involves a commitment to ongoing self-reflection and adjustment. As circumstances evolve and personal priorities shift, individuals are empowered to reassess their habits and make intentional adjustments. This adaptability ensures that these habits remain relevant and supportive of an individual's evolving needs.

In essence, encouraging lifelong habits for improved health and well-being is a transformative journey that involves tailoring health practices to individual preferences, introducing changes gradually, addressing holistic well-being, emphasizing balanced nutrition and physical activity, and fostering adaptability. By embracing these principles, individuals lay the groundwork for enduring health habits that enhance their overall quality of life and contribute to a lifelong journey of well-being.